Work Safe

An Employer's Guide to Safety and Health in a Diversified Workforce

Editorial Team:

Peter Rousmaniere, author
Stacy Burnsed, Broadspire coordinator
Matt Longman, Concentra coordinator

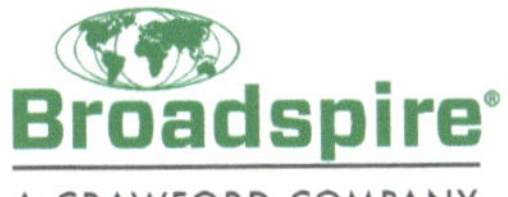

Sponsors:

Broadspire, a leading international third-party administrator, provides risk management solutions designed to help clients improve their financial results. Broadspire offers casualty claim and medical management services to assist large organizations in achieving their unique goals, increasing employee productivity and reducing the cost of risk through professional expertise, technology and data analytics. Broadspire's industry-leading medical bill review, pharmacy programs, physician review services and preferred provider networks mean further savings to you. With Broadspire, both your company and your employees get the care they need. With effective claims adjustment and thorough case management, Broadspire can have a positive impact on your employees and your bottom line. That's the difference passionate performance can make. As a Crawford Company, Broadspire is based in Atlanta, GA, with 85 locations throughout the United States. Services are offered by Crawford & Company under the Broadspire brand in Europe, including the United Kingdom. www.choosebroadspire.com, www.Broadspire.eu, www.BroadspireTPA.co.uk

Concentra, a subsidiary of Humana Inc., is a national health and well-being organization delivering effective health care solutions with innovative technology platforms, patient-first focus and clinical excellence. As a leader in consumer health care services, the company offers an expansive destination for great medical care with primary and urgent care services, physical therapy, occupational medicine, and preventive care and wellness services. With its exceptional patient experience, more than 320 national medical centers, 270 workplace health clinics and direct-to-the-patient services, Concentra is improving America's health, one patient at a time.

Free copies of Work Safe are available at
Concentra: http://www.concentra.com/education/health-library.aspx
Broadspire: http://crawfordandcompany.com/media-center/publications.aspx

For multiple bound copies, contact: Broadspire_info@choosebroadspire.com

Editor: Joni Cole. Graphic Illustrator: Bill Bedard. Designer: Sue Casper Designs. Interior Photographs by Earl Dotter, www.earldotter.com. Pages 4, 18, 26, 38
The author is grateful for the many individuals whose insights and support made this guide possible.

Table of Contents

This is only a guide and not to be relied on as legal advice.

Among members of the
foreign-born labor force in
the United States, about
half came to this country
before 1994. About 40
percent are from Mexico and
Central America, and more
than 25 percent are from
Asia.

Source: Congressional Budget Office

Yes, You Can Keep Your Foreign-Born Workers Safe!

No one has to tell you, protecting your culturally diverse workforce from injury is a big responsibility. When it comes to on-the-job safety the challenges are many, the issues complex. As an American employer, what are you legally required to do? What are the most effective ways to train a diverse workforce in safety practices? How do you deal with language barriers? How do you avoid cultural miscues? How do you get all your workers to make reducing the risk of injury a top priority?

The good news is, you have a lot of resources on your side, starting with innovative employers across regions and industries. Safety and medical professionals are spreading the word about smart practices within their professional communities. OSHA (Occupational Safety and Health Administration) has funded many projects to develop specialized safety training resources, drawing upon labor organizations and research centers. If you search for them, know-how on work safety, medical care of injured workers, and best translation and interpreting practices are out there.

Safety First. Recovery Fast.

But here's the thing. We know you want to do everything you can to maximize worker safety and injury recovery for employees with language and cultural barriers that may increase the risk of injury and complicate medical care. But we also know you don't have endless hours to devote to this issue. So that's where we come in. We've created this guide as a handy, one-stop resource of information, answers, ideas, and the most effective training methods for minimizing the risk of worker injury on the job. We highlight how to find expertise you need. We point out regulations, both in place and emerging. In addition, the back of this guidebook offers an industry-specific directory of online safety training materials designed for foreign-born workers.

The rise—and risk—of foreign-born workers

Foreign-born workers:

Year	% of U.S. population	% in U.S. workforce	% of work injuries*
1980	6.2%	6.7%	8%
1990	7.9%	9.3%	12%
2000	11.1%	12.5%	15%
2010	12.9%	16%	20%

*estimates

Whether your personal realm is in human resources, safety, medicine, insurance, public service law, or elsewhere, regardless of where you live in the United States, let this guidebook be your go-to resource. Our goal, just like yours, is to

The U.S. draws upon foreign-born workers more intensively than all other large-population nations in the world.

keep all workers injury free, and safely back to work after an injury. We sincerely hope this fast, easy-to-follow booklet serves as both a time-saver and, most importantly, a life-saver for you and your valued employees.

As a group, these workers are at greater risk of work injury than U.S.-born workers, even if they are working the same jobs. Here's why:
- Limited experience
- Language communication barriers
- Less formal education
- Cultural differences

When employers and employees don't speak the same language, the need for customized safety training is obvious, but keep this in mind: Even foreign-born workers who seem fluent in English may also be at higher risk and require specialized training. Here's why:

- The worker's frame of reference for safety expectations may differ from that of comparable U.S.-born workers. The worker's country of origin may not inculcate in its workers an expectation that safety is a high priority, and that the worker can legally demand a safe workplace.

- He or she may be unaware that in the United States employers and safety professionals are required by law to comply with many government safety requirements.

- Regardless of the level of spoken English proficiency, the worker may have very limited capacity to read English and to complete written tests at the conclusion of training sessions. A frequent glitch in training programs is that the tests are in writing, and may not have been converted to oral tests.

Given these realities, it pays to beef up safety training and injury response methods that are known to work well in diverse workforces. Throughout this guide you will find information and advice to best customize your safety training, injury response, and medical care to manage cultural and language diversity.

Make sure all your employees, including

"Hispanic" or "Latino"? Relax. They mean the same to almost everyone.

those most at risk, remain as injury-free as possible on the job, and are medically treated to return to work safely and quickly.

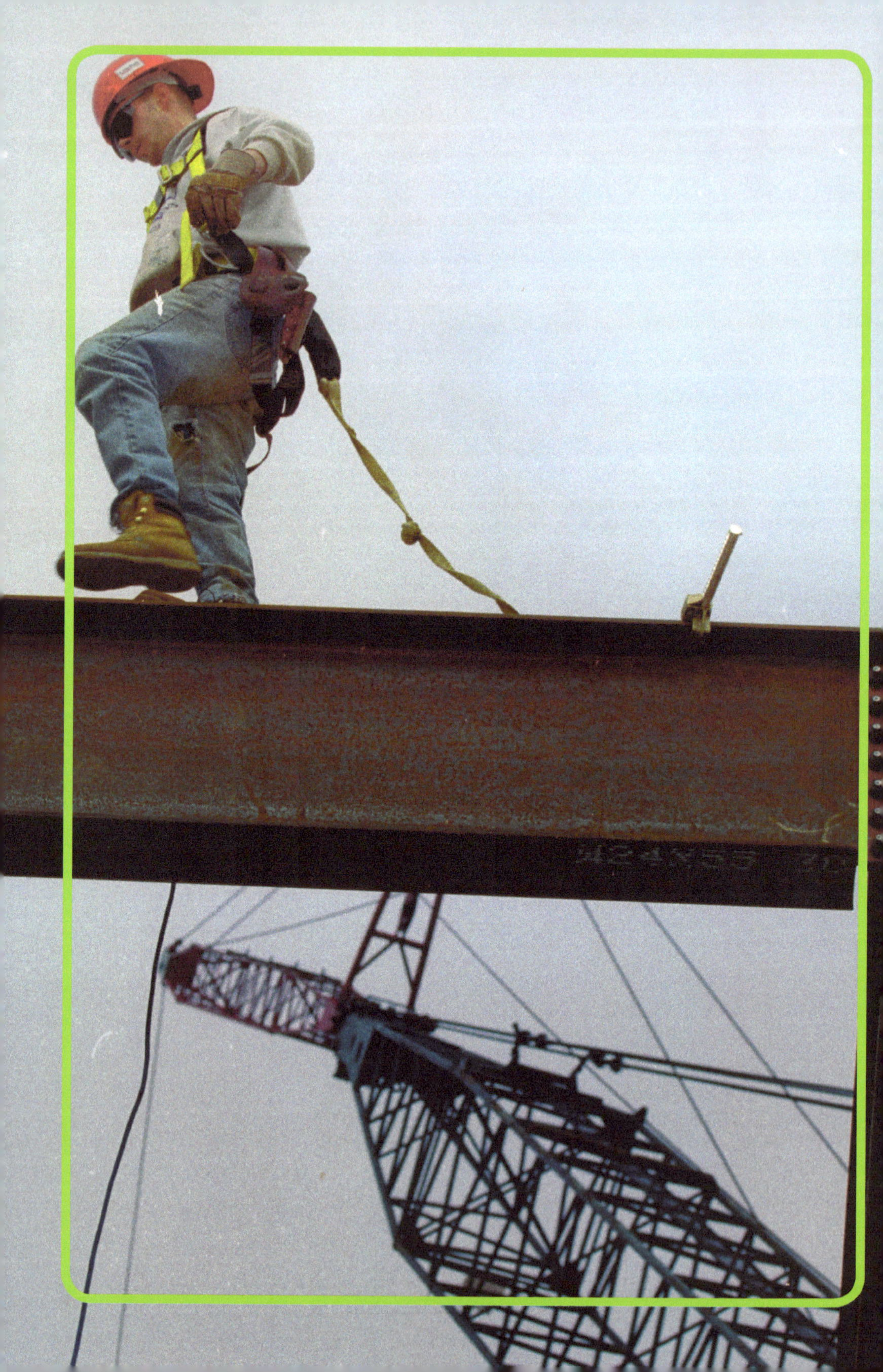

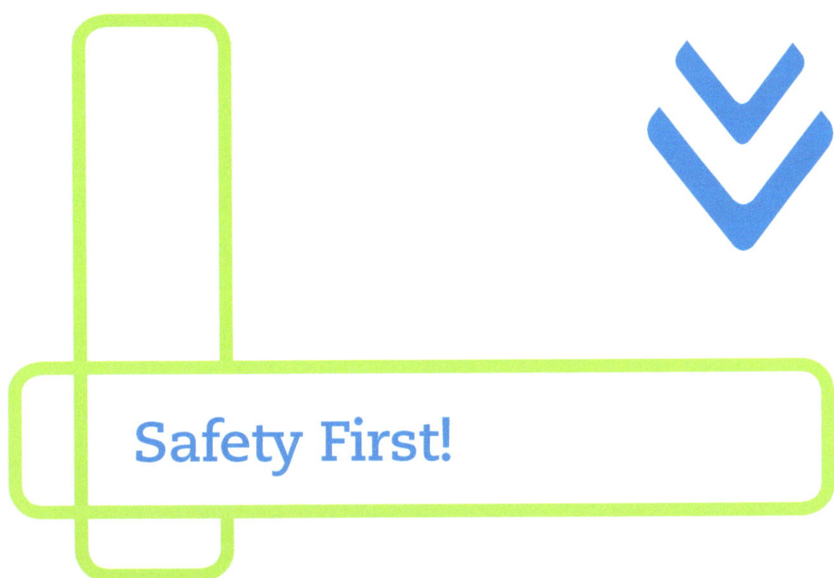

Safety First!

If you're part of a national trend, your company has seen a surge of immigrants in your workforce, especially in the past ten years. In fact, one in six workers in America was born overseas. That translates to 25 million men and women from all over the world who now work hard to make a living—and a life—in America.

In particular, moderately or low-skilled immigrants working in jobs of average or above-average injury risk are likely to face greater safety issues even if they work alongside U.S.-born workers.

Don't be taken by surprise. Even English-speaking immigrant workers are at higher risk and require specialized safety training. Why? Regardless of the level of spoken English proficiency, the worker may have limited capacity to read English and to complete written tests at the conclusion of training sessions.

In addition, because safety standards vary across countries, immigrant workers may not have the same frame of reference as U.S.-born workers. They may not expect safety to be a high priority. They may not know they have a right to legally demand a safe workplace, and that United States employers and safety professionals are required by law to comply with many government safety rules and regulations.

Given these realities, it pays to beef up training methods that are known to work in diverse workforces. Throughout this guide you will find information and practices that will help you customize your safety training to make sure all your employees, including those most at risk, remain as injury-free as possible on the job.

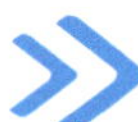

Post This:

A Summary of Safety

The following paragraph offers an easy-to-understand explanation of the basics of Safety Rules. This summary is not a substitute for required safety-related postings or documents, but it does provide good language for clear communication. Here, we've provided an English and Spanish version.

Work Safety Rules

You need to learn and obey the safety rules of your job, for your protection and for your loved ones who depend on you. You have a legal right to a safe workplace. There is a federal agency called OSHA, which stands for the Occupational Safety and Health Administration. It has studied the ways in which you can be hurt while working. The agency issues rules for safe working conditions. The rules cover things like fire hazards, falls, and dangerous materials. OSHA can inspect worksites. Safety trainers teach how to work safely. Make sure to talk to your trainer and your supervisor about any safety worries. It is your right to report any injuries and safety hazards. Your loved ones want you to work safely!

Normas de Seguridad

Tiene que aprender y obedecer las normas de seguridad de su trabajo, para su protección y la de sus seres queridos que dependen de usted. Usted tiene derecho legal a un lugar de trabajo seguro. Hay una agencia federal llamada OSHA, que son las siglas de la Administración de Seguridad y Salud Ocupacional. Esta ha estudiado las formas en que puede hacerse daño mientras trabaja. La agencia pone reglas para asegurar condiciones de trabajo seguras en todo el pais. Las reglas tienen que ver con cosas como riesgos de incendio, caídas y materiales peligrosos. OSHA puede inspeccionar los lugares de trabajo. Los instructores de seguridad enseñan cómo trabajar de manera segura. Asegúrese de hablar con su instructor y su supervisor acerca de cualquier preocupación sobre seguridad. Es su derecho reportar cualquier lesión y los riesgos de seguridad. ¡Sus seres queridos quieren que trabaje con seguridad!

Hazard Signs: Time for a Change

Workers at some five million American workplaces make or handle hazardous materials. OSHA already requires you to alert workers to these hazards and the proper way to use the materials. According to safety professionals, however, a

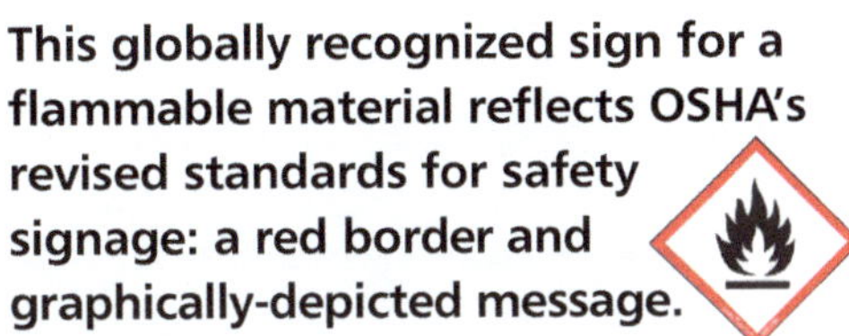

This globally recognized sign for a flammable material reflects OSHA's revised standards for safety signage: a red border and graphically-depicted message.

lot of hazard signage could be more effective, as evidenced by too many cases of missed or misunderstood messages, sometimes with fatal results.

Recently, member countries of the United Nations agreed on a new set of universal hazard signs with two key objectives: to make sure the message is understood and remembered. OSHA is introducing these signs now.

Learning to Speak the Same Language

According to OSHA, "If an employee does not speak or comprehend English, instruction must be provided in a language the employee can understand. By the same token, if an employee's vocabulary is limited, the training must account for that limitation."

To help overcome language issues, look for help with translations from bilingual employees in your workforce. Or you could hire an interpreter or a bilingual individual who may not be a safety professional, but is versed in safety training. (The chapter, Translate This!, offers tips on translators.)

The American Society of Safety Engineers advises, "Training should always be delivered in the native language of the student when possible." If not possible, follow these guidelines:

- Ensure that the student is fluent enough to understand the course material.

- For instruction and exercises, pair a less fluent student with a fluent bilingual individual.

- Avoid the use of colloquialisms or local expressions. For example, an expression like "up a creek without a paddle" may not be meaningful to someone not fluent in American English.

- Evaluation instruments, such as tests, may need to be orally administered. (A frequent glitch in training programs is that the tests are in writing, and may not have been converted to oral tests.)

- Training materials should be as visually oriented as possible. For example, use a picture of a respirator in conjunction with the word.

- Workers should be able to demonstrate recognition of warning signs and state the intended message.

- Responsible persons must determine that the individual does not represent a safety hazard on the job to himself or others.

Culture Miscues: When OK Is Not OK

It's one thing to find an interpreter who speaks the same language as an employee, but quite another to make sure he or she is also a good cultural fit. You will want to make sure the translator or trainer has a basic knowledge of local cultures and respects the differences, especially because common expressions and gestures among Americans may have very different connotations in another culture. For example, the "okay" or thumbs-up gesture used in a positive way in the U.S. translates to an offensive sign in the Middle East.

Case in Point: Trail of Tears

Cultural challenges in safety training may be hard to overcome while keeping compliant with American anti-discrimination standards. An employer learned about culture differences the hard way when it engaged a bilingual professional with training experience to conduct some safety classes. The problem was that workers for one series of classes, all men, threatened to walk out because the trainer was female, plus she spoke in a dialect that the men could understand but sent a message of condescension.

The employer replaced the female trainer with a middle-aged man who spoke the appropriate dialect. It then ran into another roadblock because the male workers prohibited the use of a mature man to train their spouses working in other assignments at the company. Eventually the employer learned that the only acceptable trainer was a male who spoke a particular dialect, and who was younger than age 30.

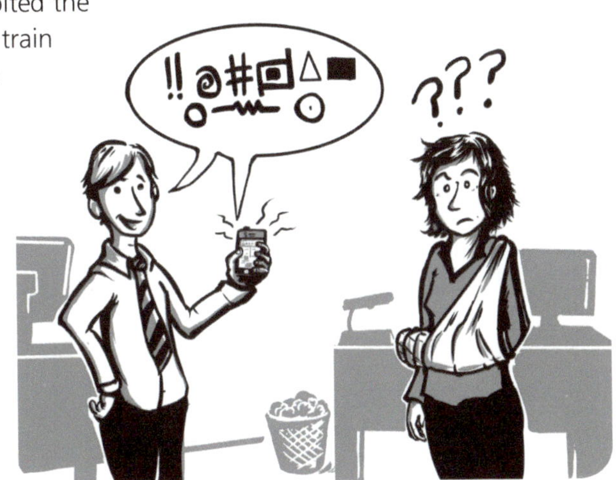

Hands Down, Hands-On Learning Works Best

Studies show interactive safety training is three times more effective than more passive learning methods in which workers are simply handed or told information. When employees are engaged in the training process and need to do more than just listen or read, they show greater knowledge acquisition, and, most importantly, accidents, illnesses, and injuries decline.

Interactive techniques for successful safety training

True case studies give the trainees the means to reflect upon the experience of other workers. Trainers can use case studies from the same industry to familiarize workers to hazards they may not have directly experienced.

Role playing enables workers to resolve a specific problem that already exists. Role playing is energizing, stimulates discussion, and is especially useful in raising awareness about hazards.

Peer training builds on the respect already accorded to seasoned workers. It also facilitates one-to-one training.

Risk mapping gathers workers into small teams to create a schematic drawing of their workplace, including major machinery, processes, entrances, exits, etc. Using different colored markers, participants note the specific hazards they identify in each area, associated with each process, machine, etc.

Body mapping, similar to risk mapping, allows participants to identify work-related health symptoms through graphic representation. Trainees are divided into small groups and given an outline of the human body, on which they place dots indicating where their body is most challenged. This reveals common patterns of functional demands that need attention.

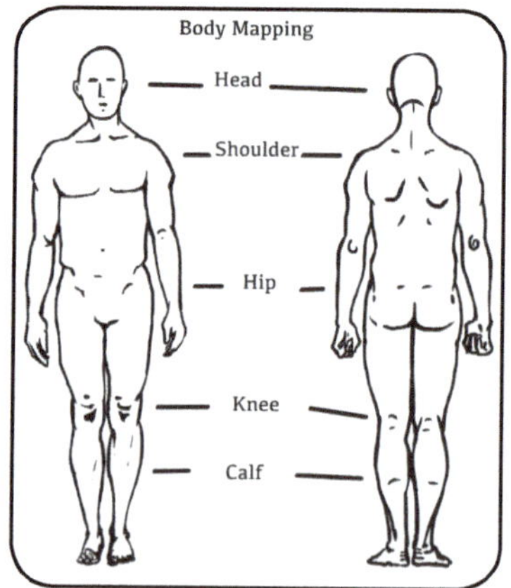

Scenarios are carefully designed and acted out scripts, designed to teach specific steps in managing hazardous situations, including what to do after an injury.

Quizzes and games reinforce training more effectively than straightforward lectures and handouts. Workers choose between several answers to questions. Each question can be followed by a more detailed explanation by the trainer, and the group may be invited to discuss issues or questions that arise.

Stories: Bringing Safety to Life

By sharing fictional accounts of realistic safety situations and characters, workers are much more inclined to "get it," especially if you include descriptions of family distress after a work injury or fatality. In essence, stories achieve safety buy-in by appealing to both the heart and mind.

What follows are two sample stories that represent effective teaching tools. The first one relates to restaurant worker safety; the second story focuses on hotel housekeeping. Regardless of your industry, you can use similar storytelling techniques, as well as follow-up materials and Q&As, to reduce the risk at your workplace.

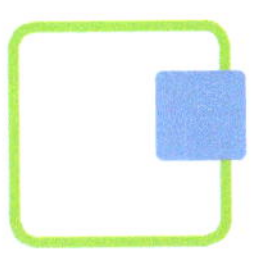

Luis works at a busy restaurant called "The Honey Pig." The dining room seats 180 people. He works at the preparation table cutting vegetables and meat all day. Part of his job is to keep the cutting machine clean.

On Monday afternoon, Luis rushes into work from his morning job as a school janitor. He needs to prepare 10 orders of vegetable servings at once and finds that his co-worker from the day shift hasn't cleaned the cutting machine.

Luis tries to quickly clean between the machine's blades by reaching in with his bare hands to pull out some remaining pieces of vegetables. The machine is not unplugged, and because the turn-on button is very sensitive he accidentally turns it on. The machine shreds his three middle fingers.

After sharing this story with workers, the trainer enhances the learning experience by following up with tip sheets for Burns and Hot Stuff, Cuts and Sharp Stuff, Slips and Falls, Ergonomics Hazards, Robberies and Assaults, Emergencies and How to Be Prepared, and Injuries on the Job. Tip sheets are ideal for brief safety meetings, which reinforce safety training over weeks and months.

Source: A Menu for Protecting the Health and Safety of Restaurant Workers

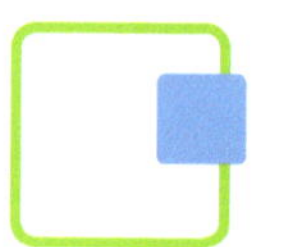

Maria recently joined her sister-in-law

to work as a housekeeper in a hotel. In her first days on the job, she found that the tools she was given by her supervisor were not as effective as the ones she uses at home and in private home cleaning, so she decided to bring to the hotel her own sprayer and squeegee. Her co-workers told her to hide them as supervisors had prohibited this practice in the past. Nonetheless, Maria continued to use her personal tools. Shortly, her dominant hand and wrist began hurting enough for Maria to report she was unable to work. An accident investigation revealed how she had violated the hotel's policies. Her supervisor was considering disciplining her.

This scenario reflects a common practice among hotel housekeepers who may insist with pride how they know best how to clean. After telling this story, the trainer engages the class in discussing how workers and supervisors can show mutual respect, praise initiative, and work safely. Maria might experiment with her tools and compare them with the approved ones. The trainer can open up a discussion of how root cause analysis may illuminate whether Maria's condition was directly related to her use of unapproved tools.

Source: A national hotel chain

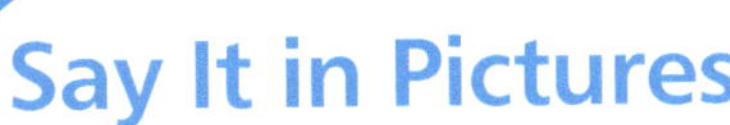

Say It in Pictures

Often the best communication about safety isn't with words but through illustrations, drawings, photos, graphics, images, and even cartoons that can bridge the language gap, and save time and confusion among your entire workforce.

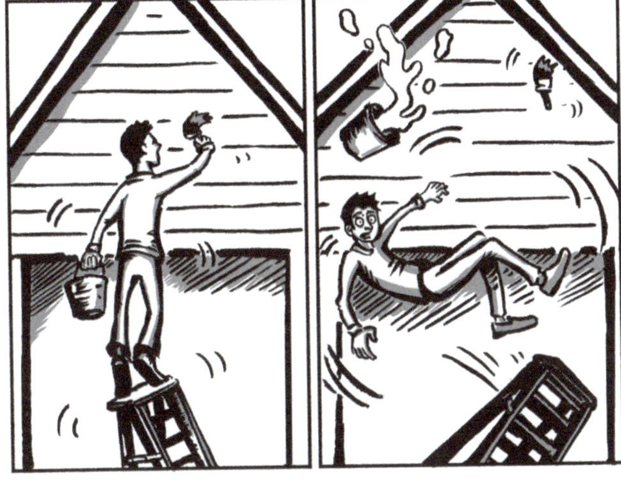

Worker safety is no laughing matter, yet sometimes a cartoon-style drawing with simple lines and concisely shown situations (as opposed to more detailed illustrations) works best to portray hazards, best practices, workplace safety protocol, and more.

In addition, safety issues in the workplace often involve movement: a fall from a ladder, an injury from repetitive motion, or a worker slipping on a wet floor. Simple drawings often prove the most effective not only for showing motion, but for indicating odor, noise, heat, or pain.

When it comes to worker safety, a picture's worth a thousand words.

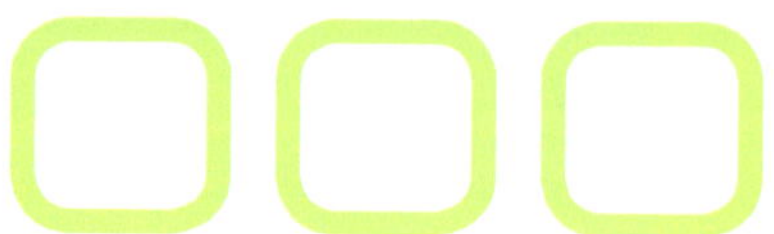

Tapping into the Network of Cartoonists

A cartoonist is an illustrator with typically a loose, simple style of drawing and a knack for telling a story in one or many panels.

Cartoonists are typically paid a one-time fee for an assignment, in which you end up with cartoons that you own. For a black and white illustration that is ¼ of a page, with four panels, per the current Graphic Artists Guild pricing and ethical guidelines, a flat fee would be $150. That works out to a pretty common page rate for pure cartooning. On a per-hour basis charges of experienced cartoonists right for these assignments will run about $60, sometimes less or more, but that will vary with the artist, of course.

You can locate cartoonists on freelance websites. They include behance. net and cghub.com. Don't be confused by highly stylized portfolio displays on these sites, as the artists are typically proficient in preparing very practical content for your purposes. You are paying for not just mechanical drafting skills, but also their talent in creating eye-catching stories.

Other freelance sites include People per Hour, Odesk, and Elance.

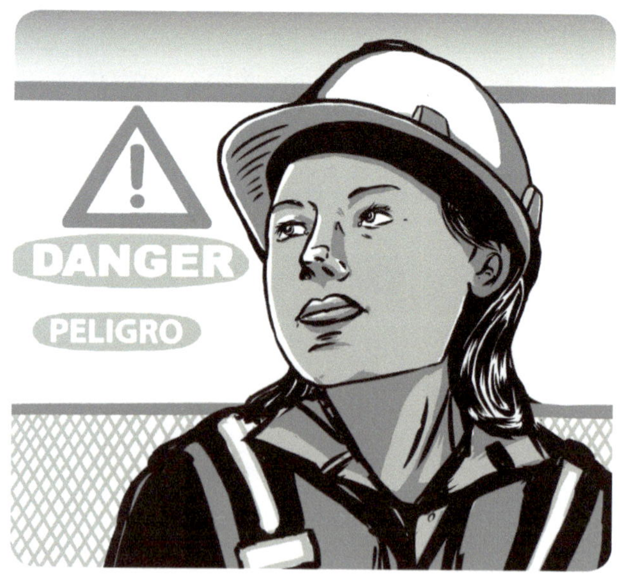

Tips for Working with Artists

- Set deadlines, building in plenty of time for review and revision.

- Peruse the portfolio. Looking through the online examples of a potential illustrator's work is essential for finding a good fit for your project. They may also have outside websites that show off more of their work.

- Don't ask for spec work. Most experienced freelancers want an official agreement before working on a job, which is only fair.

- Be specific about what you want, offering a detailed description or even thumbnails. If possible, show examples of other work that fits into a similar genre. Stay in close contact with the cartoonist as the project progresses, and offer clear feedback about what is and isn't working in each draft.

Test Your SQ (Safety Quotient)

☐ Are exposures to injuries in your workplace fully understood by a diverse workforce?

☐ Do you use written and oral exams to test workers on their comprehension of safety issues?

☐ Is your safety signage mostly graphic, with clear messaging?

☐ Is a translator or interpreter at the ready to communicate key safety messages to non–English-speaking workers?

(For each "Yes" your SQ goes up an important point!)

Free online resources. Towards the end of this guide, you'll find a list of some of the best general and industry-specific resources designed for a limited English proficiency workforce.

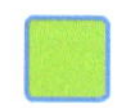

A Training Manual

Want to look at a well-conceived and executed safety manual? Find *A Menu for Protecting the Health and Safety of Restaurant Workers* on the internet.

Case Study

Glory Days Grill, a restaurant chain in the Mid-Atlantic, creates short videos with Spanish subtitles for staff training. Accessible by mobile devices and at work, the videos cover everything from food handling safety to burn prevention and seasonal menu updates.

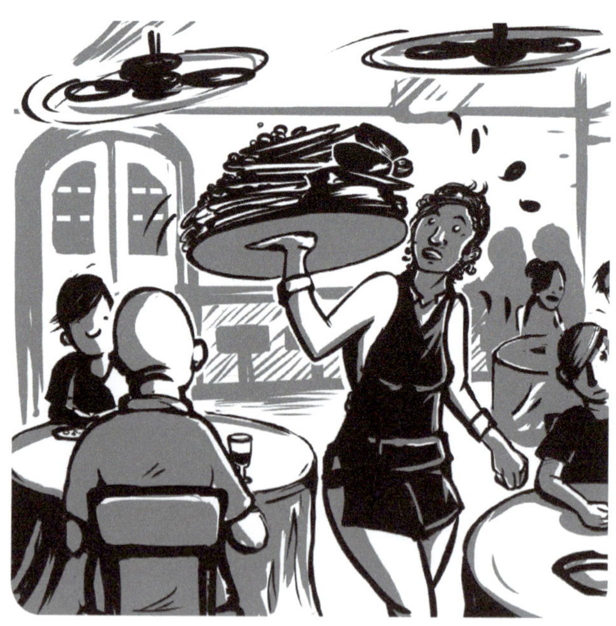

Currently, more than 60 percent of all iron and rebar workers, and more than 30 percent of helpers to brickmasons, carpenters and pipelayers are immigrants.

Source: Brookings Institution

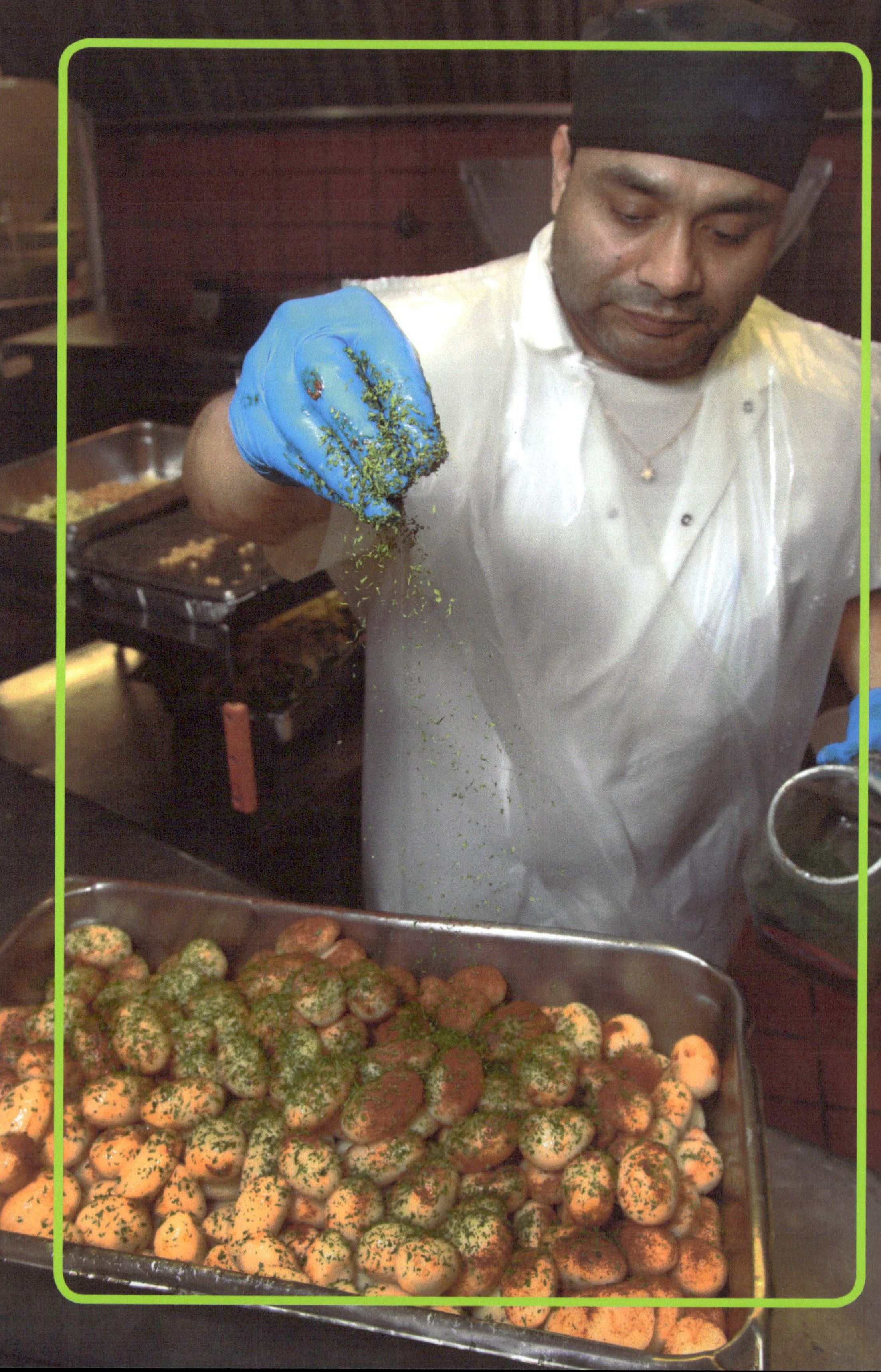

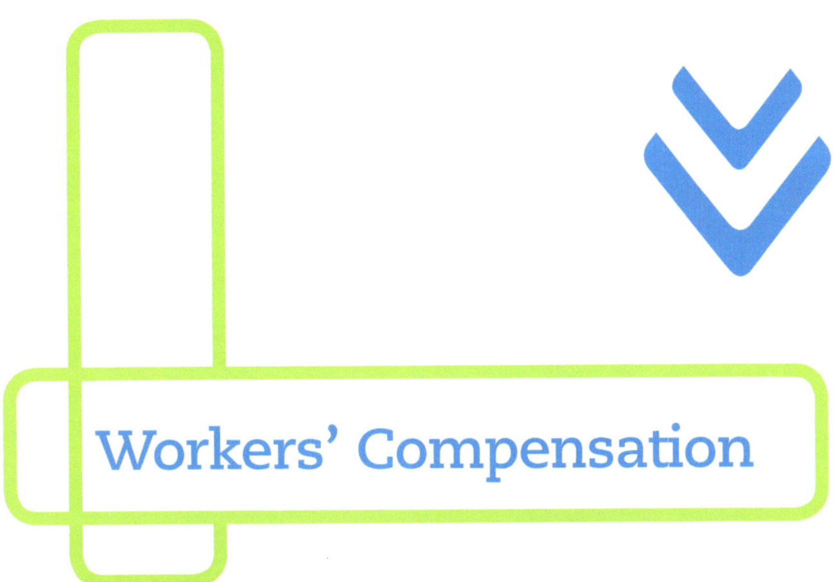

Workers' Compensation

While we don't know exactly how many foreign-born workers, or workers with limited English proficiency, file compensation claims today, the numbers are definitely rising since the 1990s. In particular, claims are increasing among workers in jobs with a serious risk of injury.

Of course, workers' compensation system benefits are equally available to any worker whose job is covered, regardless of nationality or even legal work status. One worker might speak an unfamiliar language. Another worker might not have read any of the safety instructions for his job. The best claims professionals know that each case is as individual as the worker who files it. So they take each case as it comes, one by one.

Your insurer or third-party administrator needs to be alert to what can derail claims from foreign employees: the worker's lack of understanding of the "system"; language barriers; misadventures in medical care; and myriad issues including the fact that many foreign-born workers do not have bank accounts. Regardless, all claims should be managed with equal attentiveness.

Many claims adjusters work accounts with immigrant workers who speak little to no English. In some cases, these workers are afraid to report claims for fear of being fired. Others are not sure how to report claims. There are also claimants who are familiar with the system, but file questionable claims and seek attorneys immediately. These issues and others can all result in delays. In addition, medical care can be delayed as workers are not sure where or who to go to for treatment and follow-up appointments.

States are increasingly attentive to issues involving immigrant workers, from the underground economy to the legal right to use translators.

Case Study

An immigrant worker was hospitalized at a major teaching hospital after falling down an elevator shaft and sustaining multiple severe injuries. After two surgeries, he was discharged on blood thinners and several other medications. The hospital prided itself on its state-of-the-art "academic" medicine in a "patient-centered" atmosphere.

The hospital discharge unit gave him a stack of papers in English (he spoke no English) with instructions on how to call two separate outpatient clinics for follow-up appointments. It loaded him up with prescriptions without any instructions on where he should go to get them filled. He had no money for bus fare, much less to pay for the medications.

Make sure to assign a qualified individual to provide coaching. Someone on blood thinners could develop a life-threatening hemorrhage.

One Navigator Is Not Enough

Many employers and claims organizations assign a specially designated individual with bilingual skills to certain injured workers. This solo navigator fix can work to some extent, but can't be expected always to prevent or resolve the messy complications that often arise after a work injury occurs. An injured worker may be competent in English in a workaday sense and still her case can present challenges for claims management.

For example, low-income foreign-born workers often work second jobs. They may be responsible for carpooling other employees. They may rush headlong to return to work in fear of being laid off. They may even wish to return to their country of origin to get medical care or recover from an injury. And their expectations for workers' comp benefits may not be well grounded.

Talk with your insurer or third-party administrator about how you can jointly anticipate and respond to these challenges. Inventory the cultural and linguistic diversity among your employers. Match that with worksite, adjuster, and case manager resources. Jointly identify medical providers who can be most helpful. Jointly review written communications about workers' comp benefits and worker obligation to make sure they are free of jargon.

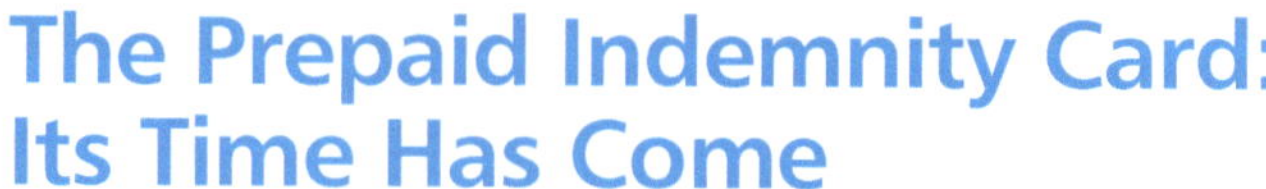

The Prepaid Indemnity Card: Its Time Has Come

Approximately 15 percent of adults in America don't have bank accounts. But for people who earn less than $30,000 a year that number jumps to about one-third being "unbanked." Why the dearth of bank accounts? Sometimes it's a preference; other times the pressure of dealing with a financial institution can be intimidating. Regardless, people who do not have bank accounts can easily pay hundreds of dollars a year in check-cashing charges.

The good news: an increasing number of employees receive their wages via a payroll debit card. Thus, they don't need to set up a bank account for direct deposit, or incur check-cashing charges. This raises the question: why can't injured workers have access to a similar solution, and get their benefits via a prepaid card?

The answer, in concept, is that they can. The claims payer would contract with a debit card vendor with a service customized for workers' compensation claimants. The vendor sends the card to the claimant, with information about which ATM machines will honor the card. At one of these ATMs, the claimant withdraws some or all of the indemnity benefits available at that time, without incurring a transaction charge. The claimant thereby avoids cash-checking fees and has access to cash 24/7.

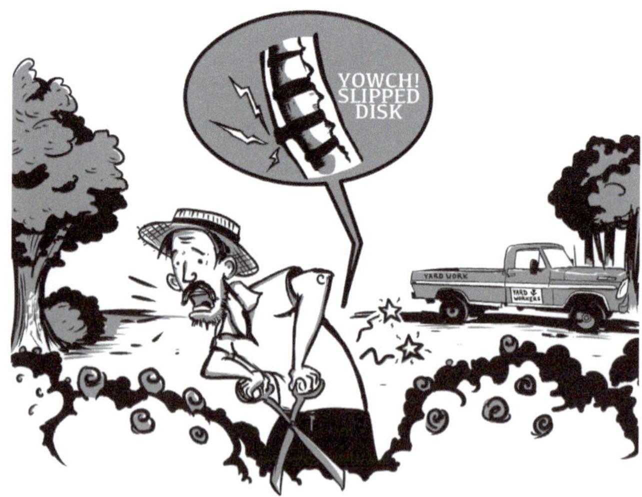

State regulators, the banking system, and insurers are trying to remove roadblocks preventing the use of prepaid indemnity cards, but widespread implementation of such a process has been slow going. This method of payment needs to give claimants access to multiple ATM machines without incurring charges. In addition, the process needs to address other technological challenges, and meet state standards on insurance payments.

Ask your insurer or third-party administrator when (not if) they plan to introduce these cards.

In Plain English (or Somali, or Portuguese)

Most written summaries of workers' comp benefits are hard to understand by persons with limited English skills or little experience with the American ways of employee benefits. If your workforce is covered by workers' comp (in all likelihood it is), here is a summary that might work for you and your workers. It's presented in English and Spanish.

Workers' Compensation

If you get hurt at work, or you get sick from your work, workers' compensation insurance pays for the medical treatment you need and will pay you part of your average weekly wage if you cannot work. You do not have to pay anything to get workers' compensation. Your employer by law must provide it and you have a right to it if you are hurt at your job. It does not matter whether the accident was your fault, another worker's, or your employer's, you still get the same benefits. The law says you cannot sue your employer or co-workers for extra money because you believe they caused your injury.

Make sure to tell your supervisor of your injury as soon as possible. If your injury or illness developed gradually, report it as soon as you learn or believe it was caused by your job. Your employer will then send an injury report, which you sign, to the insurer.

Reporting an injury immediately helps avoid delays in receiving medical care and benefits.

You are expected to do everything you can to get healthy and to return to work when your doctor says you can. Please respect your doctor's instructions. The doctor may say that you can return to work but with restrictions.

Note: The workers' compensation laws are different in each state.

Indemnización por accidentes de trabajo

Si se lastima en el trabajo o se enferma debido a su trabajo, el seguro de compensación por accidentes de trabajo paga por el tratamiento médico que necesita y pagará parte de su salario semanal promedio si no puede trabajar. Usted no tiene que pagar nada para obtener la compensación por accidentes de trabajo.
Por ley su empleador debe darlo y usted tiene derecho a esta compensación si se lastimó en su trabajo. No importa si el accidente fue culpa suya, de otro trabajador o de su empleador, usted obtiene los mismos beneficios. La ley dice que no puede demandar a su empleador o compañeros de trabajo por dinero adicional aunque crea que le hayan causado la lesión.

Asegúrese de reportar su lesión lo antes posible a su supervisor. Si su lesión o enfermedad se desarrollaron de manera gradual, reportela tan pronto se entere o crea que fue causada por su trabajo. Su empleador envía un reporte de lesión, que usted firma, a su asegurador.

Reportar lo mas antes posible ayuda a evitar una espera larga para la recepción de beneficios, como la atención médica.

Se espera que haga todo lo posible para recuperar la salud y regresar al trabajo cuando su médico lo autorice. Por favor respete las instrucciones del médico. El médico puede indicar que puede regresar a trabajar pero con restricciones.

Las leyes de compensación por accidentes de trabajo son diferentes en cada estado.

This is only a guide and not to be relied on as legal advice.

Percentage of total population
who speak a language other
than English at home:

12.3%   Spanish and Spanish
        Creole languages

2.9%   Asian and Pacific
        languages

3.8%   Other languages

Source: Census Bureau

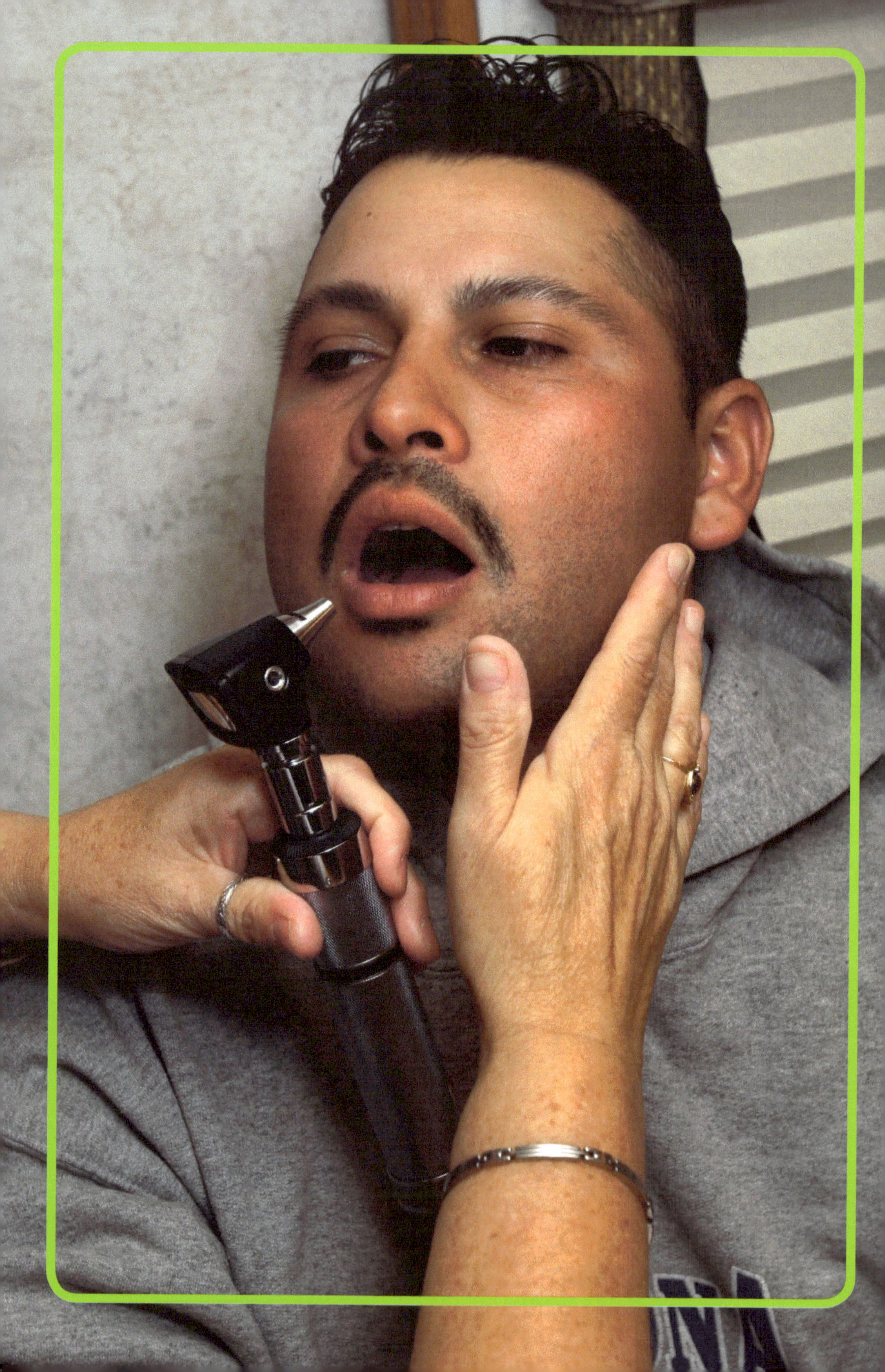

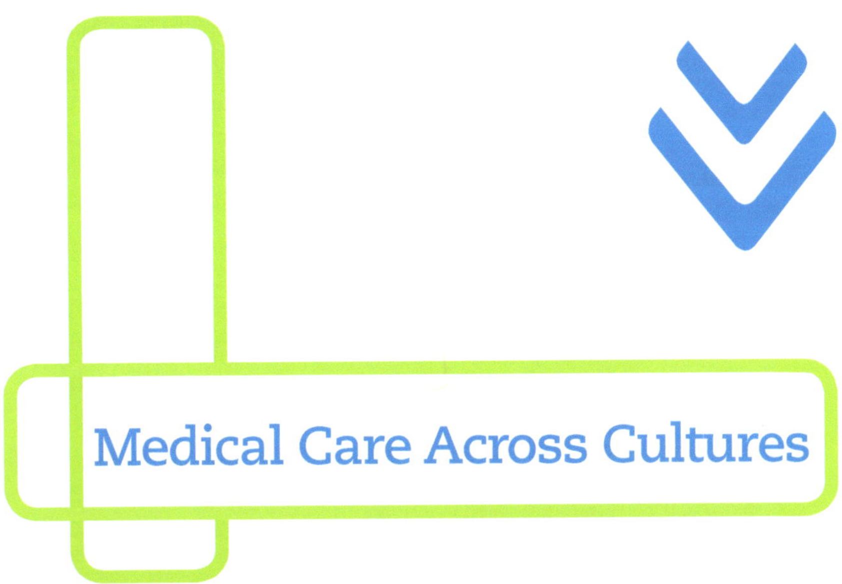

Medical Care Across Cultures

The goal is straightforward—to keep all your workers healthy and productive. In the unfortunate event of a worker injury or job-related illness, you want your employees to receive the best available medical care possible, and to assure a safe and expedited return to work.

But what isn't so straightforward is the best way to help your medical providers deliver that care, especially to a diverse workforce. When treating people from different countries and cultures, healthcare professionals face three main challenges that all too often lead to a series of medical mishaps:

Triple Threats to Quality Cultural Care

1. Lower health literacy. Health literacy is the degree to which individuals can obtain, process, and understand basic health information and services needed to make appropriate health decisions. Health literacy affects what people know about diseases, how they use the healthcare system, if they understand medical instructions, and if they adhere to these instructions.

Healthcare professionals commonly experience low health literacy among many foreign-born individuals. Limited health literacy causes people to have trouble using everyday health information—available both inside and outside the doctor's office—to confront situations that involve life-changing decisions about their well-being.

This is a problem throughout America, especially common among foreign-born individuals.

2. Cultural Miscues. Even workers who seem fluent in English may still adhere to health beliefs and practices from their country of origin that are dissimilar, or at direct odds, with Western care. Culture influences how a person defines a health problem and whom (and how) they expect to treat it. For example, the Chinese concept of disharmony is corrected not only by harmony in health, but also good weather and good fortune. Other cultural traditions can lead to self-treatments that complicate or discredit the care provided by a Western medical professional.

3. Limited English. The English language is rife with idioms ("draw blood", "back on one's feet") and other challenges to communication with workers who are not proficient in English. Whether it's an inability to communicate basic health information, or a failure to convey or understand the essence of an exchange, language barriers are often one of the main causes of disappointing medical outcomes.

For even the most committed and talented healthcare professionals, cultural discrepancies often remain a mystery…and a source of frustration. What may seem like an obvious medical fact—the scientifically proven cause or cure of a health condition, the way the body works, or the diagnosis of certain symptoms, for example—may not conform to an immigrant worker's traditional views. A case in point: in some societies, it's believed that coughs are always fatal. In addition, excellence in care can mean something dramatically different to patients of different backgrounds.

In the past, few if any nurses, doctors, wellness professionals, health advocates, or medical case managers received training in or methods to address poor health literacy, cultural miscues, and low English proficiency. What they learned, they learned on the job, which left too many patients falling through the cracks.

Fortunately, the healthcare community now recognizes the crucial importance of helping medical personnel overcome barriers and improve working relationships and outcomes for diverse patient populations, including those serving in your company. Today, it's widely recognized that medical knowledge is no longer enough. Caregivers have to go beyond simply addressing the language gap with the help of a translator or medical interpreter (which is no easy task in and of itself). To succeed in this era of health care demands both linguistic and cultural sensitivities, awareness, and knowledge.

Immigrants historically have been three times more likely than native-born Americans to be uninsured for health care. This has complicated access to care.

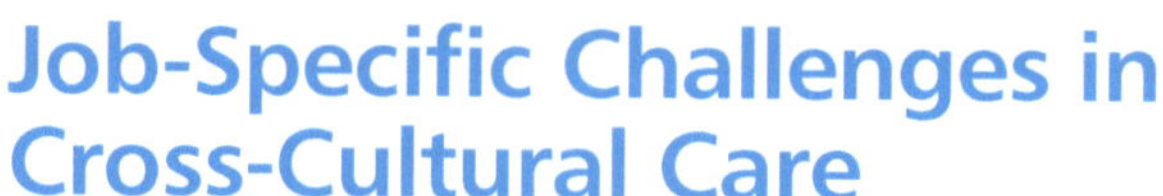

Job-Specific Challenges in Cross-Cultural Care

Onsite health professionals often have to work hard in coaching for-eign-born workers on wellness programs, safety awareness, and best ways to return to work after injury. They may have more pressing concerns. They may view Fate as overruling their personal freedom of choice as far as their safety and health. When an injured worker returns to work with restrictions, nurses may need to be especially diligent to make sure the worker is complying with those restrictions.

Physicians may be treated with undue deference and seen as "all knowing" by patients who then feel cheated if they are not given a specific diagnosis with immediate treatment. Doctors may have to compensate for incomplete or inaccurate information both on written forms and in oral interviews. They may order fewer or more diagnostic tests for patients because they don't understand or believe the patient's description of symptoms. They may need to be more attentive to the patient's ability to follow treatment instructions, and address the common attitude: Why both-er the doctor for a follow-up visit if the health problem has resolved?

Medical case managers are likely to have to confront a patient's steep learning curve when it comes to understanding the American healthcare system. As with everyone who serves as a healthcare resource, case managers need to respect their clients' beliefs and customs, for example the reliance on traditional healers in some cultures. In relation to loved ones who may support patients with advice on treatment, even the question: "Who is family?" isn't always straight-forward, given the answer may include unconventional kin, godparents, and other non-blood relatives.

Occupational health nurses, as a profession, are acutely aware that low literacy skills of workers lead to higher incidence of injuries, illnesses, and fatalities. They know how low occupational health literacy leads to non-compliance with education and training, failure to ask questions and respond, flawed histories of injury, illness or health concerns, and delayed accident reporting.

Side Effects of Low Health Literacy, Cultural Miscues, and Language Barriers

- Lack of reliable medical records from the patient's past

- Failure to seek preventative care, leading to more emergency room visits and hospital admissions

- Patient's inability to articulate medical history and concerns, and describe presenting symptoms

- No written agenda for medical visits

- Possibly significant errors when trying to comply with medication/follow-up instructions

- Possibly unreasonable expectations of what should or should not be included in care (for instance, expecting some sort of medication to be dispensed every visit, regardless of the diagnosis; or, insisting on X-rays, MRIs, or other testing when it is not indicated)

- Missed appointments

- Lack of follow-through with lab or imaging tests, or ignoring referrals to consultants

- Misuse of medications

- Less effective management of chronic diseases, such as arthritis or high blood pressure.

- Difficulty navigating the healthcare system, from filling out forms to locating providers and services

Talk with your preferred medical providers. Show them a copy of this chapter.

The Rewards of Knowing the Risks

The better workers understand the risks of their job, the more likely they are to avoid injury. In addition, the more workers are aware of the symptoms related to those risks, the more likely they are to report those symptoms to medical providers, and thus benefit from preventative or timely treatment.

It may seem surprising, but low risk awareness isn't just an issue among workers from other countries with different sensibilities about safety. Even many native-born workers do not accurately recognize some of the potential dangers on the job, and hence fail to or delay reporting symptoms that may be related. That's why it's important for your employees' healthcare providers to nurture risk-awareness within your entire workforce. Here are a few simple but key questions medical providers should be asking workers:

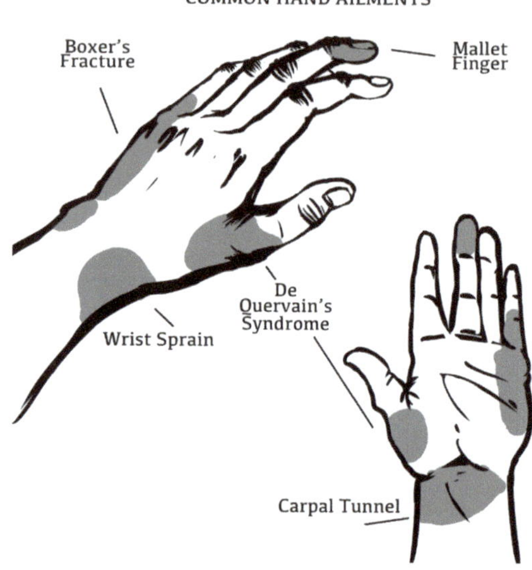

• What do you do for work? Please describe in detail.

• Are you exposed to anything at home or work that you are concerned about? For example, high heat, chemicals, noise, fumes, dust?

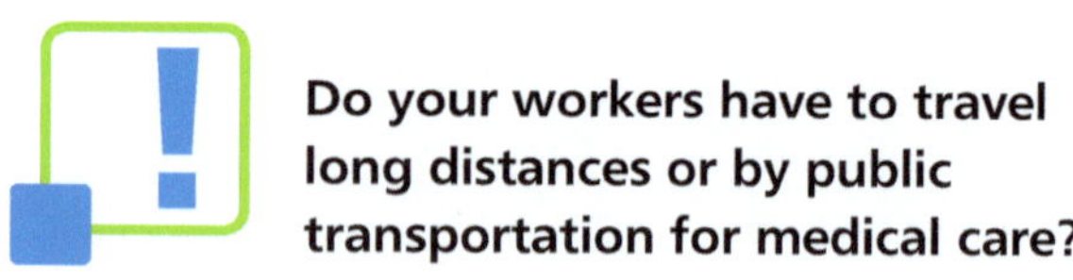

Do your workers have to travel long distances or by public transportation for medical care?

Caution: Kid Translators = Compromised Care

It's a familiar scene. A non–English-speaking patient arrives at the doctor's visit with a family member, friend, or bilingual fellow employee who is there to help with translation. The interpreter may even be the patient's child. While this may be common practice it is fraught with pitfalls that can compromise care. One study found that family members who serve as translators misinterpret a quarter to half the questions asked by physicians. These ad hoc interpreters also often fail to ask important questions about issues like drug allergies or the proper use of antibiotics. They may confuse the doctor's orders, or refuse to convey questions about sexually transmitted diseases and illicit drug use.

While it may seem convenient to use a bilingual employee or relative to interpret when medical care is being delivered to a non–English-speaking worker, most are not qualified to translate important health or safety-related information with a reliable degree of accuracy. Quality translation and interpreting requires not just a fluency in both languages, but a mature awareness and respect of cultural nuances, and strong problem-solving skills. For interpreting, the individual must be able to work under pressure and have command of any special glossary of terms that come with the subject matter.

The interpreter must also be aware that patients sometimes see them as their advocate, but their job is to be a neutral intermediary, not to champion the patient's cause. The translator also may have to deal with the healthcare provider's lack of patience due to time constraints, making it more difficult to give patients the attention they deserve, for example to make sure all instructions are understood.

Young children and adolescents are never appropriate interpreters. Friends, family members, and co-workers of the patient can make mistakes in interpreting, or try to advocate for the patient instead of acting as a neutral party.

The Joint Commission on Accreditation of Hospitals says "it is not appropriate to rely on untrained individuals as the primary source for bridging communication barriers during medical encounters with individuals who are deaf or speak a language other than English."

Rx for Hospital: Pro Medical Interpreters

Because accurate health information is so vital to keeping your workers safe, and because medical discussions often involve difficult terminology, specialized interpreters are key to successful patient care…but only if they do a quality job. One study of medical clinics showed a high rate of substantial errors or omissions in interpreting, including complete failure to translate key items. In addition, the interpreters often engaged in speech unrelated to interpretation.

In 2009, less than half of the hospitals in the U.S. had formal policies regarding the use of minors, friends or family, or non-trained staff as interpreters. Today, hospitals, outpatient clinics, and work-site health programs are more aware of the risks of relying on non-professional medical translators, and are playing catch-up in terms of making interpreting services available, affordable, and trustworthy. Some have started training programs on basic interpreting skills for volunteers and non-clinical staff members. Others avail themselves of outside medical interpreters who work either on site or over the phone, a necessity in communities that lack bilingual nurses, doctors, and other direct care givers.

The Civil Rights Act obligates medical providers to arrange for patient communication in the most suitable language for the patient.

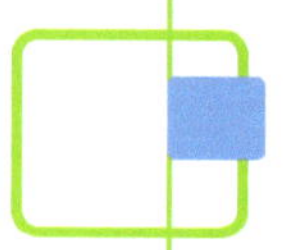

TIPS FOR
Overcoming Language Differences

- Slow down. Plan double the normal time.

- Use active listening.

- Avoid using family members as interpreters on medical issues.

- Use plain, non-medical language.

- Seek reputable websites with information in other languages (for instance spineuniverse.com/español and Healthyroadsmedia.org).

- Show or draw pictures.

- Always look at the patient, not the interpreter.

- Limit the amount of information provided, and repeat it.

- Produce easy-to-read written materials with translations.

- Confirm the patient's understanding of your message.

- Avoid legalese in conversation and documents.

- Do not let the patient feel judged or ashamed at their lack of English.

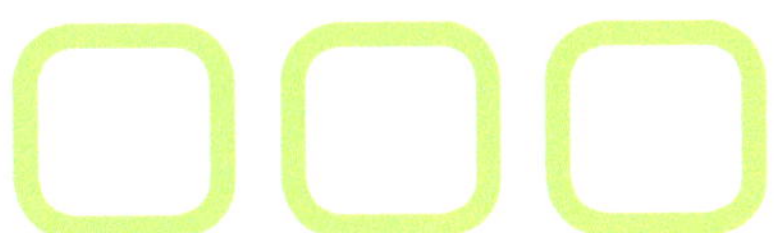

Test your cultural awareness.

> **Do you** recognize and accept that individuals from culturally diverse backgrounds may desire varying degrees of acculturation into the dominant culture?

> **Do you** understand that age and lifecycle factors must be considered, such as high value placed on the decision of elders, the role of eldest male or female in families, or roles and expectations of children within the family?

> **Do you** recognize and understand that beliefs and concepts of emotional well-being vary significantly from culture to culture?

> **Do you** respect that customs and beliefs about food, its value, preparation, and use are different from culture to culture?

Adapted from "Promoting Cultural and Linguistic Competency: Self-Assessment Checklist for Personnel Providing Primary Health Care Services."

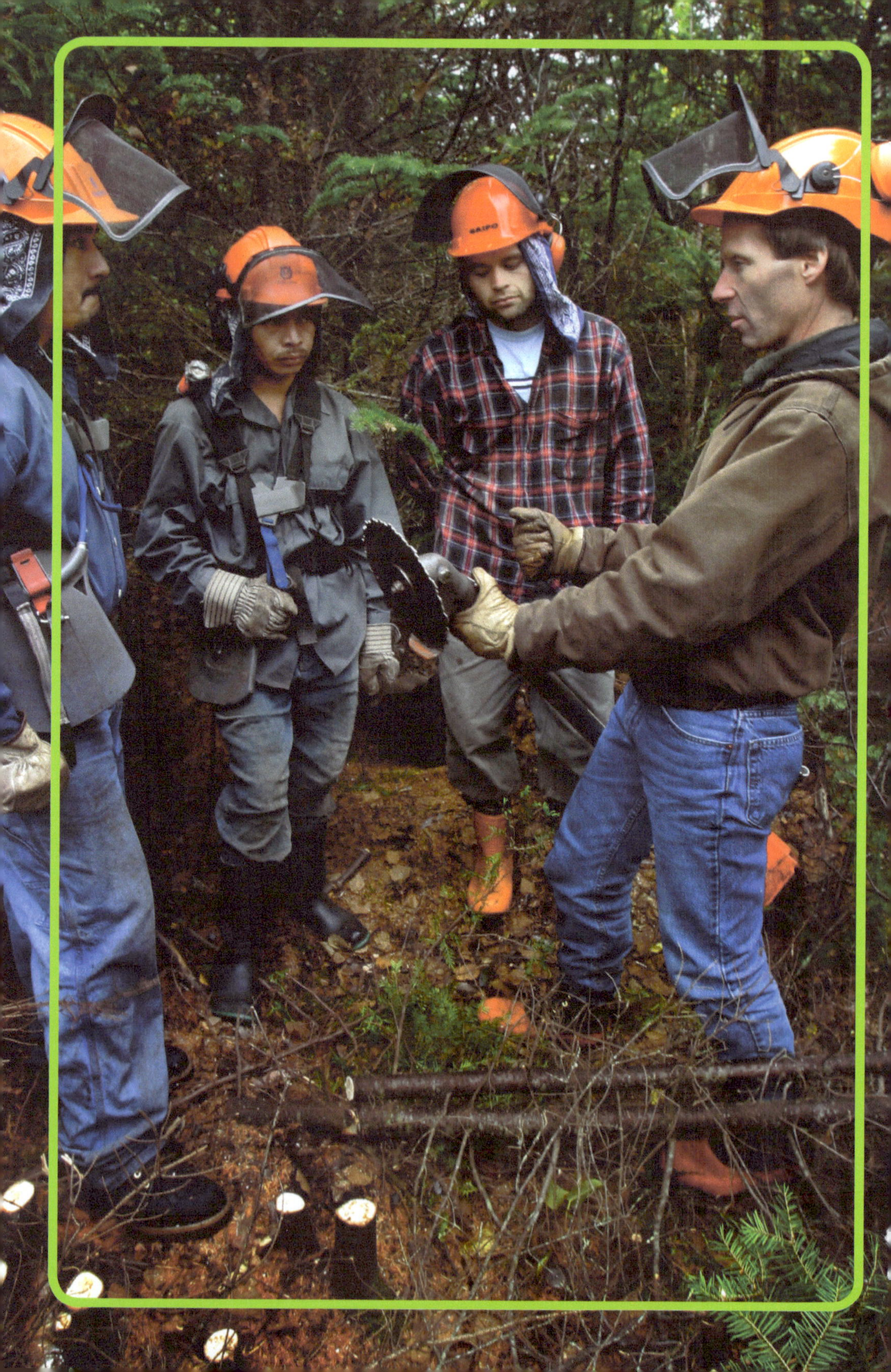

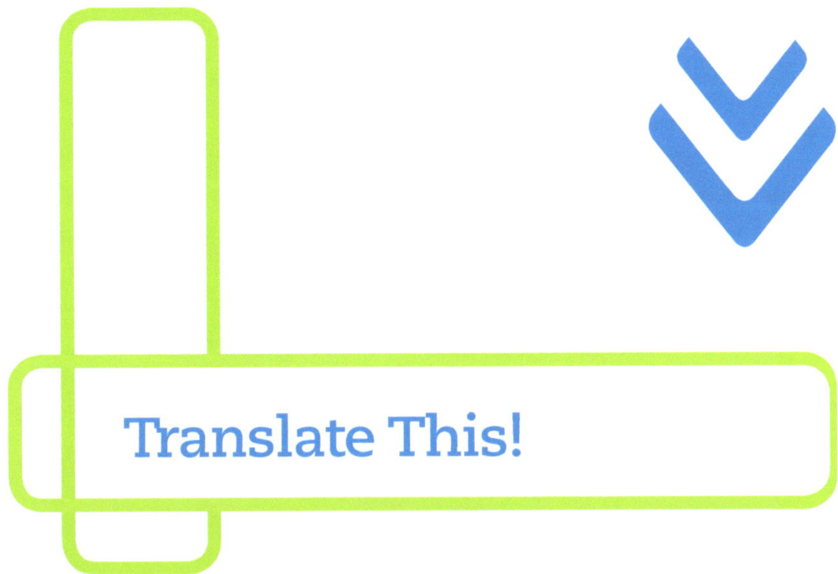

Translate This!

Earlier parts of this guide touched on the importance of translation and interpretation (TI) to overcome language barriers that can contribute to a higher risk of injury and illness. This chapter delves into the art of TI, how to engage TI resources, and how to sidestep pitfalls.

What do interpreters interpret? More than words, it's meaning. The goal is to have the listener understand the message as if it were heard directly from the original speaker. Quality interpreting reflects cultural terms, expressions, and idioms that have bearing on the meaning of the content. Translators work bi-directionally, going back and forth between two languages.

Given the diversity of today's workforce, TI services benefit companies in each of the following areas:

- **employee orientation**

- **work safety training**

- **communication of employee rights and duties**

- **responding to work injuries**

- **receiving workers' compensation benefits, and safe return to work**

Technology-Based Translation: Don't Trust It

Talk into a smartphone. A free mobile app will quickly translate your statement into a language of your choice, both in writing and by voice. You can also go online to Google Translate or iTranslate, paste in written content, then read a translation. For instance, you might say, "Are you exposed to anything at home or work you are concerned about?" A few moments later, a translation will appear. The person to whom you are speaking might answer, "Yes, I work with chemicals that smell bad and sometimes I feel funny. My boss said I have to wear a mask and gloves, but sometimes there aren't any available."

Only here's the rub: you can't always count on accuracy. **Consider the following examples of what we found when we put these tools to the test in several languages:**

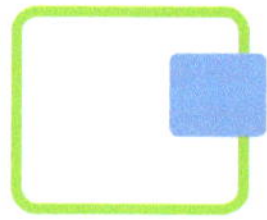

English: **"You are sick at work."**
Spanish: **"You are sick of your work."**

English: **"You were injured."**
Spanish: **"You were wounded."**

English: **"Make sure to tell your supervisor of your injury as soon as possible."**

Mandarin: **"Make sure to tell yours yours injury, as soon as possible supervisor."**

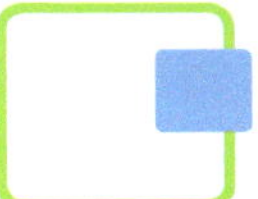

English: "The workers' compensation laws are different in each state."

Google Translate: "The workers' compensation laws are different in each country."

Bing: "The workers' compensation laws are different in each status/condition."

The American Society of Safety Engineers advises, "Training should always be delivered in the native language of the student when possible."

» Live Interpreters: A Better Choice

Rather than rely on technology and its foibles, it's much better to avail yourself of human-based interpreting services. Below is an explanation of two types of these services, each appropriate for specific tasks.

Telephonic interpreting is appropriate for a task such as an accident analysis or post-injury return to work consultation. This is called consecutive translation, when the interpreter listens, then speaks the other language.

(Simultaneous translation typically involves the use of headphones, as at international conferences.)

The employer places a request by phone; the telephonic service typically responds very quickly. The call is put on a speaker phone or the phone is passed between the parties.

Interpreting vendors are introducing live two-way video interpreting, to allow the interpreter to see the subject's gestures.

On-site interpreting. The demands of interpreting during safety training may justify using an on-site rather than telephonic interpreter. An on-site interpreter can read body language, establish trust, and decipher facial expressions. Many cultures are very expressive, and the unspoken tells just as much as the words. Before translating, the interpreter should learn any special glossary of terms that may be used.

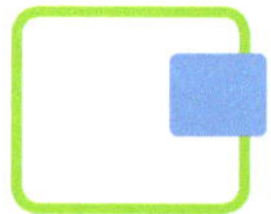

Evolving Legal Requirements

The trend is patchy but undeniable: government agencies and private employers are increasingly being required by law to interact with employees and their customers in the language most suitable for effective communication. Additional requirements are likely to follow, and professions such as human resources, safety, and medical care have been upping their efforts to provide instruction and service delivery in a language their employees and customers can understand.

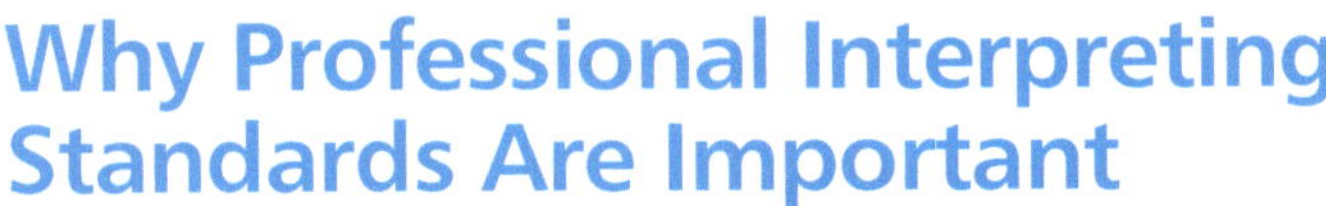

Why Professional Interpreting Standards Are Important

Fortunately, there is a trend toward more caution in using non-professional interpreters. While there is no generally accepted nationwide "gold standard" certification for interpreters or translators, the American Translation Association does offer a generalized certification program. There are also special certifications available for medical translators. And to re-emphasize, without question, hiring a highly experienced, even certified, translator is the smartest, safest route.

An Overview of Standards

Accuracy: Nothing should be omitted or added. The tone and spirit of the source language message should be retained.

Non-Advocacy: The interpreter/translators should not be put into the role of advocate for anyone.

Courtesy: They should be culturally competent, sensitive, and respectful.

Confidentiality: They should not divulge any information obtained through their assignments.

Proficiency: They should disclose when they are unable to accurately perform their assignment.

(Adapted in part from Language Interpreter and Translator Code of Professional Conduct)

Case Study

An English-speaking hospital staff once mis-interpreted a patient's complaint of "intoxicado" as an admission of being intoxicated, not that the patient felt nauseous. The mistake resulted in permanent paralysis and a multi-million dollar financial settlement.

Applying your employees' skills

A possible alternative to hiring an outside professional is to use a bilingual employee — with a big caveat. He or she must be trained!

Hospitals, under the gun by accrediting agencies, are sending more of their volunteer interpreters to training courses, some receiving up to 50 hours of classroom work. Several national training programs, such as Bridging the Gap at www.xculture.org, are available for those wishing to improve their skills in medical interpreting so that it is culturally and linguistically appropriate.

It is not hard to test an employee's TI skills. Language Testing International, affiliated with the American Council on the Teaching of Foreign Languages, can conduct a short test by phone. If you expect to test bilingual employees often, you might arrange for a freelance translator to be on call, also by phone. In any event, prepare a few paragraphs of text representing a typical conversation, including specially used terms. Ask the employee to immediately translate it. The professional translator then grades the effort on a scale demarcating a "pass" threshold. At least one testing firm is introducing a proficiency test for an individual to take on her or his own initiative, to get a special certificate.

One evaluator (for a Polish translation) summed it up:
"There were numerous errors with regard to grammar rules, omissions, word choices, to mention a few. And quite often a general style of translation was weird."

The Golden State: Taking the Lead in Translation

Not surprisingly, California leads the country in prescribing translation and interpretation. In 2011, 35% of its civilian workforce was foreign born, compared to 16% nationwide. About half are naturalized citizens.

California's Senate Bill 853, which became effective in 2009, requires health insurance organizations in California to provide free and timely translation and interpretation services for patients with limited English proficiency. The bill essentially requires all California insurance companies to be responsible for their own "language assistance program" to meet state requirements, but without undue burden on the company. They must also collect, summarize, and document all information on enrollees' language needs as garnered from surveys.

The California Division of Workers' Compensation in 2012 issued regulations requiring the use of a qualified interpreter during medical appointments of injured workers if the patient cannot effectively communicate with his or her treating physician because he or she cannot proficiently speak or understand the English language.

Sources for TI Professionals

For the employer with only occasional need for TI, one approach is to retain a freelance professional. The American Translation Association has an online directory of its members. There are many state and sub-state-specific associations that can be located by searching for "translation associations [name of jurisdiction]," such as "translation associations Iowa." In your area there may be other multi-language sources. Catholic Charities in Boston, for example, covers many languages for employers, arising out of its services for immigrant households.

Several national firms also provide interpretation in multiple languages, and may provide for translation of written materials and transportation services for injured workers. Your workers' compensation insurer or third-party administrator likely retains a service, and can be helpful in your search.

Charges for Translation Services

Cost quotes can be per word (either the source or the target document), per hour, and/or fixed sum. Telephonic interpreting on demand costs $1 - $3 per minute, governed mainly by volume and languages used. On-site interpreting costs can be quoted per hour or segment of day, with travel time separately priced, or by fixed total cost. Ask about charges in the event of last-minute cancellations, termination during service delivery, and emergency requests.

Check out Proz.com as one online source of freelance translators.

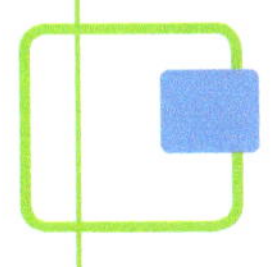

10 Planning Steps for Translation and Interpreting

1. Determine what you need: on-site safety training, telephonic interpreting, document translation, or other issues.

2. Determine the most common languages you need translated, including dialects.

3. List the departments that need translation services. Create special glossaries of terms.

4. Consider whether medical care is involved, requiring specialized translation and interpreting standards.

5. Internal resources: Create a directory of employees with a facility in languages who may be called upon from time to time.

6. Decide whether one office will be responsible for coordinating internal recruitment of staff and purchase of services.

7. Telephonic Interpretation: Estimate how often and how long an interpreter typically will be needed. Will this service be primarily requested on demand or scheduled? If scheduled, how much lead time is needed? Is two-way live video interpreting available?

8. Ask vendors for response times to requests for services and minimum qualifications of personnel to be assigned. Ask about a process for continuation of language services in the event of a disaster or emergency. Ask for references and to see a professional code of ethics.

9. Cost quotes from vendors. Ask to specify by type of service and by language.

10. Contract management. Define a process for tracking usage of language services, which party will be responsible for this, and how this data will be provided. Describe your confidentiality needs and procedures.

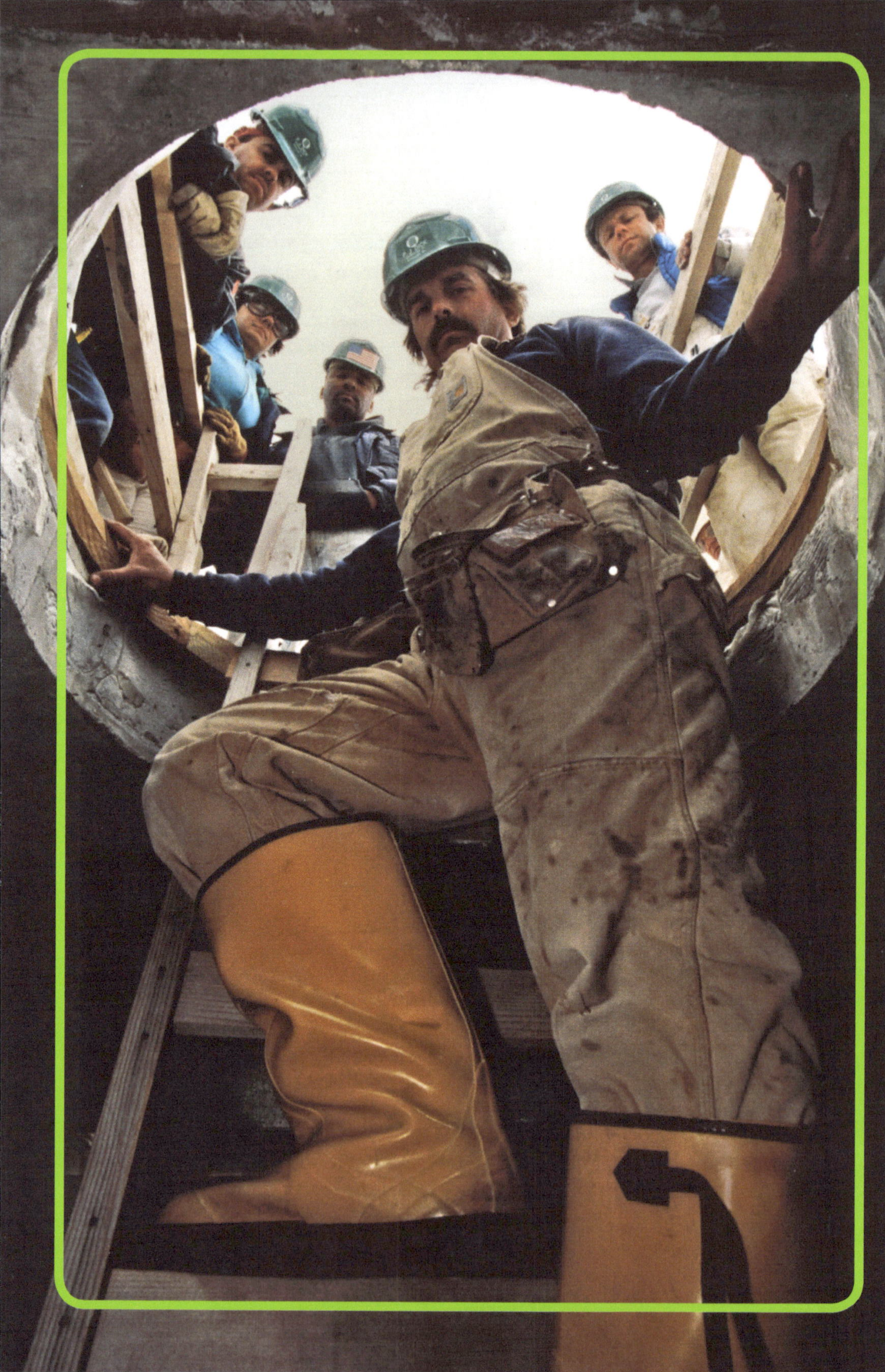

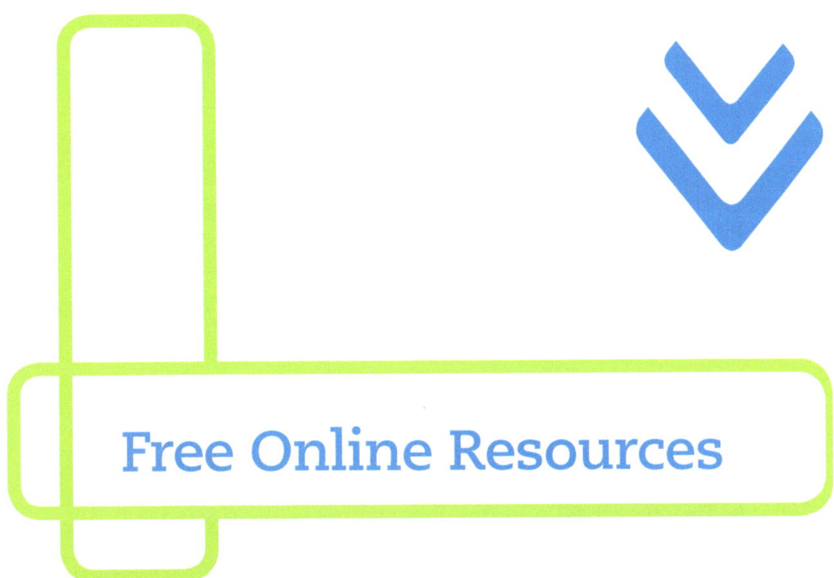

Free Online Resources

We evaluated many online resources to identify the most useful ones for organizing a safety training program for a diversified workforce. Some resources are pertinent for all industries and are included under General Resources. Others are devoted to specific industries with large foreign-born worker participation. Many can be accessed by internet search, and have English, Spanish, and sometimes other language versions.

Read guides found on the internet for ideas for your own customized guide. As a model for a guide for a diversified workforce, we especially recommend: *A Menu for Protecting the Health and Safety of Restaurant Workers Manual*, accessible by internet search.

To design an injury prevention program from the ground up, CalOSHA posts online a family of preparation tools:
http://www.lohp.org/projects/smallbusiness/laws_iipp.html

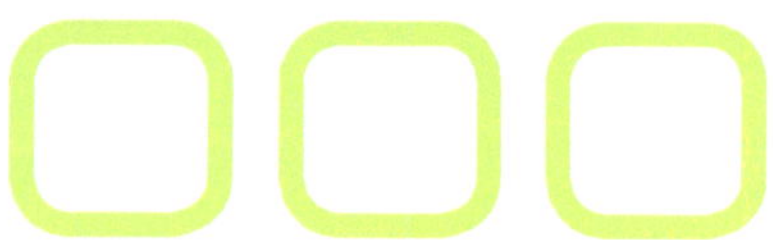

>> General Resources

California Department of Industrial Relations Cal/OSHA ergonomic publications. Training resources in Spanish and English on the subjects of ergonomics, confined space, hazard alerts, and other workplace issues. **http://www.dir.ca.gov/dosh/PubOrder.asp**

New York State Insurance Fund. Safety Posters. Simple posters with just a picture and a few words, to reinforce safety training. Spanish: **http://ww3.nysif.com/SafetyRiskManagement/SpanishResources/ SPSafetyPosters.aspx**

OSHA. Compliance Assistance Quick Start: Hispanic Outreach A starting point for employers with Spanish-speaking workers, with links to many OSHA resources. **http://www.osha.gov/dcsp/compliance_ assistance/quickstarts/hispanic/index_hispanic.html**

OSHA en Español. A dedicated website for assistance in Spanish. instruction.**http://www.osha.gov/as/opa/spanish/index.html**

OSHA Harwood Grant materials. Harwood Grant-funded safety training tools covering many industries. Most are available in a language other than English. **http://www.osha.gov/dte/grant_materials/material_listing_topic.html**

State Compensation Insurance Fund of California. Safety Meeting Topics. Many training tools designed for work breaks or before the shift. In English and Spanish. **http://www.statefundca.com/safety/ safetymeeting/SafetyMeetingTopics.aspx**

State Compensation Insurance Fund of California. Safety Videos. Most available in Spanish. **http://www.statefundca.com/safety/SafetyVids.asp**

State Compensation Insurance Fund of California. Tailgate Topics. Over 100 tailgate trainings designed for work breaks and start of shift meetings. English and Spanish. **http://www.statefundca.com/safety/ safetymeeting/SafetyMeetingTopics.aspx**

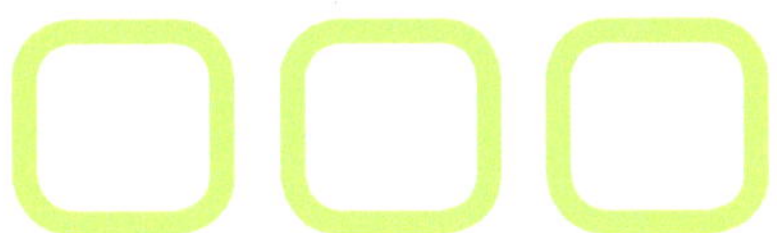

University of California at Berkeley, Labor Occupational Health Program Center for Occupational and Environmental Health. Multilingual Health and Safety Resource Guide. The only comprehensive catalog of web-based safety training resources for non–English-speaking workforces. Organized by topic and language, and periodically updated.
http://lohp.org/docs/library/multilingualguide4th.pdf

UCLA Labor Occupational Safety and Health. Resources and Publications. Of note is **The Worker's Sourcebook: La Fuente Obrera,** a compilation of simple Spanish-language materials for workers.
http://www.losh.ucla.edu/losh/resources-publications/index.html

New Jersey Department of Health. Right to Know Hazardous Substance Fact Sheets. More than 1,600 fact sheets have been completed, over 900 translated into Spanish.
http://web.doh.state.nj.us/rtkhsfs/factsheets.aspx

Oregon OSHA. Peso Training Resources Program. Many topics covered in hour-long presentations and tailgate versions. Spanish.
http://www.cbs.state.or.us/osha/educate/peso.html

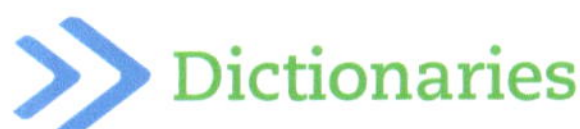 ## Dictionaries

OSHA. Dictionaries (English-to-Spanish and Spanish-to-English). Prepared by OSHA's Hispanic Task Force. Over 2,000 general OSHA, general industry, and construction industry terms.**http://www.osha.gov/dcsp/compliance_assistance/spanish_dictionaries.html**

Oregon OSHA. English-Spanish Dictionary of Occupational Safety and Health Terms. A large, specialized English-to-Spanish dictionary of terms used in worker safety, such as "wash your hands" and "imminent danger."
http://www.wellnessproposals.com/safety/handouts/englishspani.pdf

The Southwest Center for Occupational and Environmental Health. English/Spanish Glossary.
https://sph.uth.edu/research/centers/swcoeh

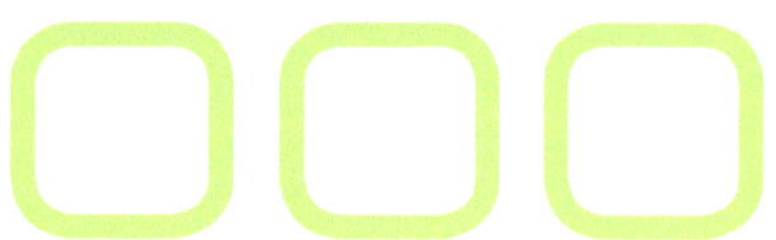

Resources for selected industries

Note: URL cited may be for an English version of a document. Spanish and other versions are usually available.

Agriculture

General Agricultural Safety
AgSafe: Agricultural Safety Training Materials. National Ag Safety Database. **http://nasdonline.org/document/2125/d000101/ agsafe-agricultural-safety-training-materials.html**

Field Workers – pesticides
Association of Farmworker Opportunity Programs. Project LEAF (Limiting Exposure Around Families) materials**. http://www.epa.gov/ oppfead1/cb/csb_page/updates/2013/project-leaf.html**

Field Workers – heat illness
Water. Rest. Shade. The Work Can't Get Done Without Them. OSHA. **http://www.osha.gov/SLTC/heatillness/edresources.html**

Heat Stress: Farmworker Health and Safety. Association of Farmworker Opportunity Programs. **http://www.osha.gov/dte/grant_materials/fy09/sh-19485-09.html**

Packers and Sorters
Packing House Safety. New York State Department of Labor Hazard Abatement Board. **http://www.nycamh.com/qdynamo/download.php?docid=481**

Simple Solutions: Ergonomics for Farm Workers. U.S. Department of Health and Human Services. **http://www.cdc.gov/niosh/docs/2001-111/pdfs/2001-111.pdf**

Sanitation Workers
Nighttime Sanitation. University of Medicine and Dentistry of New Jersey, School of Public Health. **http://www.osha.gov/dte/grant_materials/fy07/sh-16627-07.html**

Textile Workers
Cotton Dust Fact Sheet.
Texas Department of Insurance, Division of Workers' Compensation.
http://www.tdi.texas.gov/pubs/videoresource/fscottondust.pdf

Garment Workers
Stretches For Garment Workers. State Compensation Insurance Fund of California. **http://www.garmentcontractors.org/Stretches_garment-Workers_Eng.pdf**

Sewing Machine Operators: Feel Better! Work Better!
California Department of Public Health.
http://www.cdph.ca.gov/programs/hesis/Documents/sewing.pdf

Spanish: **http://www.cdph.ca.gov/programs/hesis/Documents/sewingsp.pdf**

Construction Workers

General Construction Work
Health Hazards in Construction. Construction Safety Council.
http://www.osha.gov/dte/grant_materials/fy09/sh-19495-09.html

Buildsafe California Educational Materials and Publications – Tailgate Training Materials. California Department of Public Health.
http://www.cdph.ca.gov/programs/ohb/Pages/BuildSafe.aspx#conducting

EICOSH: Electronic Library for Construction Occupational Health and Safety. Large online library of training resources including images and a special section in Spanish.
http://www.elcosh.org/index.php

Seguridad en la Construcción. Georgia Tech Spanish Language Construction Training Website. **http://www.oshainfo.gatech.edu/hispanic/empieze-aqui.html**

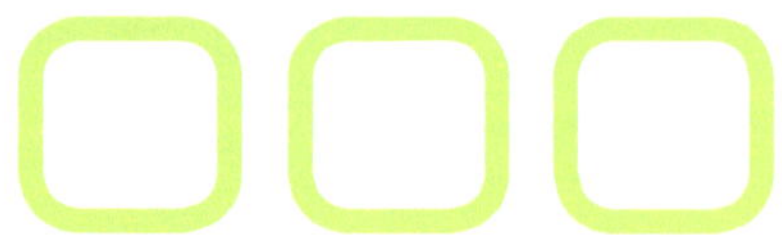

Safety Matters Construction Series. New York State Insurance Fund in Spanish. **http://ww3.nysif.com/SafetyRiskManagement/SpanishResources/SPSafetyMattersConstructionSeries.aspx**

Respiratory Protection: Training Videos. OSHA.
http://www.osha.gov/SLTC/respiratoryprotection/training_videos.html

Insulation Workers
Asbestos Fact Sheet. OSHA.
http://www.osha.gov/OshDoc/data_AsbestosFacts/asbestos-factsheet.pdf

Carpet Layers
Carpet Layer Safety. State Compensation Insurance Fund of California.
http://www.statefundca.com/safety/safetymeeting/SafetyMeetingArticle.aspx?ArticleID=375

Painters
Falling Off Ladders Can Kill: Use Them Safely. OSHA.
http://www.osha.gov/Publications/OSHA3625.pdf

Roofers
Fall Protection: Taking It to a Whole New Level. University of Alabama.
http://www.osha.gov/dte/grant_materials/fy10/sh-21006-10.html

Buildings and Grounds

Building Maintenance
Cleaning Chemicals and Your Health. OSHA. 2013. Poster is available in English, Spanish, Chinese Traditional and Tagalog. **https://www.osha.gov/pls/publications/publicationathruz?pType=Industry&pID=401**

Gardening and Landscape
Tips for a Healthy Back. National Center for Farmworker Health, Inc. 1997. **http://www.ncfh.org/pdfs/4526.pdf**

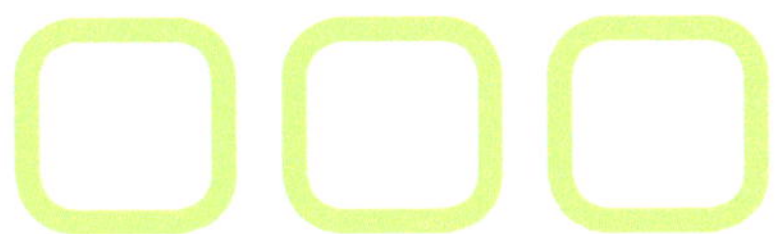

Back Injury Prevention for the Landscaping and Horticultural Services Industry. Kansas State University, Agricultural Extension. 2006. http://www.osha.gov/dte/grant_materials/fy06/46g6-ht22/back_injury_prevention.pdf

Landscapers versus Texas Critters Fact Sheet. The Texas Department of Insurance. 2012. English: **http://www.tdi.texas.gov/pubs/videoresource/fslandscapecritters.pdf**

Risk Topics: Floor Cleaning Procedures for Slip, Trip and Fall Prevention. Zurich. 2009.
http://www.moverschoiceinfo.com/res/docs/pdf/safety-handbook/floor-cleaning-procedures-for-STF-prevention.pdf

Housekeepers
Working Safer and Easier: For Janitors, Custodians and Housekeepers. California Department of Industrial Relations. 2005. https://www.dir.ca.gov/dosh/dosh_publications/janitors.pdf

Janitorial Workers
Janitorial Training Materials. WOSHTEP (Worker Occupational Safety and Health Training and Education Program). 2012. **http://www.losh.ucla.edu/woshtep/resources/janitorial-training-materials.html**

Janitorial Safety Training Guide. Labor Occupational Health Program (LOHP) at the University of California, Berkeley. 2012.
English: **http://www.dir.ca.gov/chswc/woshtep/Publications/JanitorialTrainingGuide.pdf**

Health Care

Safety Training Resources for Hospitals: Free Downloadable DWC Safety Publications. Texas Department of Insurance. 2013.
http://www.tdi.texas.gov/wc/safety/videoresources/targhospitals.html

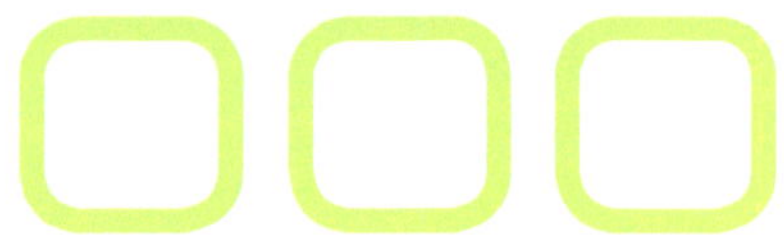

Home Health Aides

Caring for Yourself While Caring for Others: Practical Tips for Home Health Care Workers. Service Employees International Union. 2013. **http://www.lohp.org/docs/projects/homecare/homecareenglish.pdf**

Nurse Aides

Safe Patient Handling Techniques for Healthcare Providers. OSHA, Lake Sumter Community College. 2010. **http://www.osha.gov/dte/grant_materials/fy10/sh-20829-10.html**

Restaurant Work

A Menu for Protecting the Health and Safety of Restaurant Workers Manual. OSHA, University of California at Berkeley. 2010. **http://www.osha.gov/dte/grant_materials/fy10/sh-20864-10/rest_worker_manual.pdf**

Keeping the Restaurant Safe Is No Accident. OSHA, Restaurant Opportunities Centers United. 2009. **http://www.osha.gov/dte/grant_materials/fy09/sh-19478-09.html**

Dishwashers

Food Service Workers Safety Guide. Canadian Centre for Occupational Health and Safety. 2012. **http://www.ehs.uconn.edu/forms/TTT/fwsg.pdf**

Hand Dishwashing (Hot Water Sanitizing). South Carolina Dept. of Health and Environmental Control. 2008. **http://www.scdhec.gov/administration/library/CR-003159.pdf**

Cooks

Important Temperatures to Remember for Potentially Hazardous Foods. South Carolina Dept. of Health and Environmental Control. 2008. **http://www.scdhec.gov/administration/library/CR-002160.pdf**

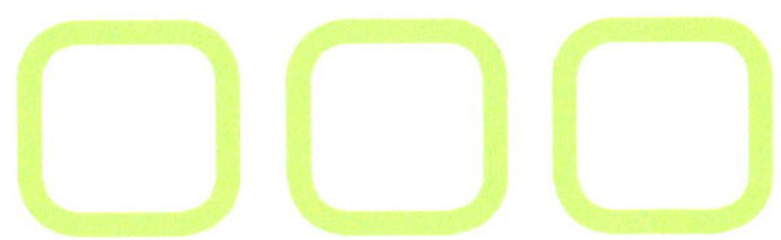

Waitstaff

Waitstaff Health and Safety. Texas Department of Insurance Division of Workers' Compensation Safety Education and Training Programs. 2013. Spanish: **http://www.tdi.texas.gov/pubs/videoresourcessp/ spstpwaitstaff.pdf**

Meatpacking

Meat and Poultry Worker Safety. OSHA, Nebraska Appleseed Center for Law in the Public Interest. 2010.
http://www.osha.gov/dte/grant_materials/fy10/sh-20833-10.html

Poultry Processing
Poultry Industry Hazards. OSHA, Telamon Corporation. 2010.
http://www.osha.gov/dte/grant_materials/fy10/sh-20835-10.html

Seafood Processing
Handling Seafood Safely. North Carolina Sea Grant. 2001.
http://nsgl.gso.uri.edu/ncu/ncuh01001.pdf

Food Processing Sanitation
Worker Training Course for Food Processing Industry Sanitation. OSHA, Georgia Tech Research Corporation. 2009. **http://www.oshainfo. gatech.edu/foodsanitation/foodsanitation-worker.html**

Other Occupations

Taxi Drivers
Taxi and Delivery Drivers Safety Sheet. Texas Department of Insurance Division of Workers' Compensation Workplace Safety. 2013.
http://www.tdi.texas.gov/pubs/videoresource/stpsmtaxi.pdf

Airline Baggage Handlers
Ergonomic Solutions: Baggage Handling. Texas Department of Insurance. 2010. **http://www.wellnessproposals.com/safety/handouts/ essibaggagehand.pdf**